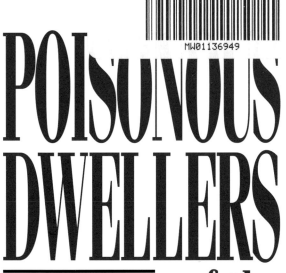

POISONOUS DWELLERS

Description ✦ Habitat
Prevention ✦ Treatment

of the

DESERT

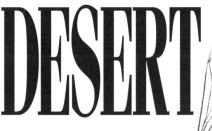

Text by

TREVOR HARE

Illustrations by

BARBARA TERKANIAN

SOUTHWEST PARKS AND MONUMENTS ASSOCIATION
TUCSON, ARIZONA

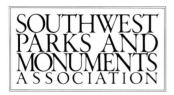

Copyright © 1995 by Southwest Parks and Monuments Association,
Tucson, Arizona 85701

Publisher's Note: SPMA records indicate that since 1960 *Poisonous Dwellers of the Desert* by Natt Dodge has been reprinted seventeen times and 300,000 copies have been sold. We cannot trace how many were in the seven printings previous to that date. It has served as a much valued reference over the decades, and one person told us she believes it saved her life.

We felt it was time to update and renew the contents, and this volume is not a new edition, but an entirely new book. We hope it will be as useful and used as its predecessor.

ISBN 1-877856-53-3

Library of Congress Number 94-69816

04 03 02 01 00 99 98 97 96 95   10 9 8 7 6 5 4 3 2 1

Editorial: Sandra Scott
Design: Christina Watkins
Production: TypeWorks, Tucson, Arizona
Printing: Lorraine Press, Inc.

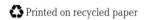 Printed on recycled paper

CONTENTS

INTRODUCTION

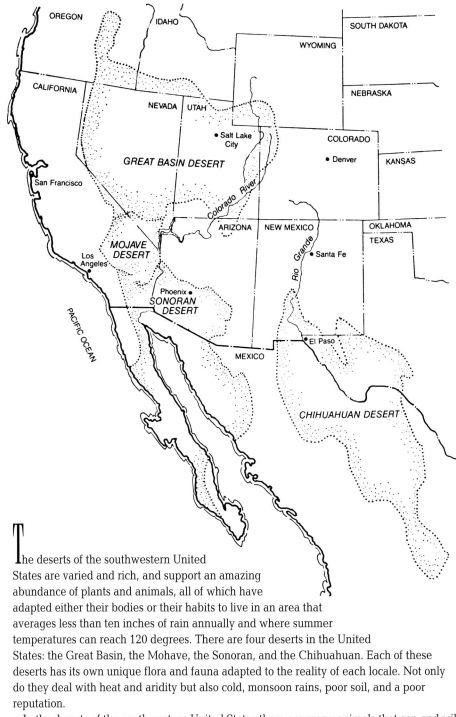

The deserts of the southwestern United States are varied and rich, and support an amazing abundance of plants and animals, all of which have adapted either their bodies or their habits to live in an area that averages less than ten inches of rain annually and where summer temperatures can reach 120 degrees. There are four deserts in the United States: the Great Basin, the Mohave, the Sonoran, and the Chihuahuan. Each of these deserts has its own unique flora and fauna adapted to the reality of each locale. Not only do they deal with heat and aridity but also cold, monsoon rains, poor soil, and a poor reputation.

In the deserts of the southwestern United States there are many animals that can and will inject or spray their venom into unwary travellers. While some of these animals, such as the gila monster, are unique to the deserts, other venomous animals are present throughout the

United States, including different species of rattlesnakes, other pit vipers, coral snakes, spiders, scorpions, and the social insects (Hymenoptera). The deserts may have a greater abundance of venomous animals because of the extended active season and the great amount of open space. Also, the unique environmental constraints of these arid regions may have caused some animals to evolve venomous adaptations in order to survive. These animals are not lying in wait except when hunting small prey. Most are non-aggressive and bite only when handled, molested or trapped.

The venomous animals in this book comprise two groups: **arthropods** (invertebrate animals with an exoskeleton and jointed body and limbs), which includes crustaceans, arachnids (spiders), and insects; and **reptiles** (snakes and lizards).

A venom is defined as a naturally occurring poison composed of proteins, enzymes and other organic compounds that can be injected into a body. It is metabolically expensive to produce and is not readily wasted. Venom is used in two ways: for defense or in prey immobilization and digestion. It may be delivered through sting, bite, or urticating hairs, although some animals are known to spray venom. The sting, employed by most arthropods, usually delivers venom with a modified ovi-depositor. The bite, utilized by the reptiles, some ants, the centipedes and arachnids, envenomates with some sort of modified teeth or fangs. Urticating hairs, used by tarantulas and puss caterpillars for self-defense, are hollow or porous hairs with a unicellular venom gland at the base of each through which venom is injected.

The purpose of this book is to identify these animals, give practical advice on how to avoid them, or how to treat their bites or stings if they occur. We hope it will also put to rest some misconceptions and help people understand these animals for what they are, creatures evolved in a specific role in nature.

First aid in this book is that recommended by the Arizona Poison and Drug Information Center in Tucson. The staff there are certified poison specialists backed up by doctors expert in venomous animal stings and bites. They provide a free service which will evaluate your bite or sting and suggest a course of action, and can assist your doctor in determining proper treatment.

Assorted people may have varying allergic reactions to the same venom. A **mild reaction** to a bee sting for one person may just be a small welt and short-lived pain. Another individual may experience a **severe reaction** which may include: burning pain and itching at the site of the wound; itching on the palms of the hands, soles of the feet, neck and groin; general body swelling; nettlelike rash over the body; labored breathing; intense pain; high or low blood pressure; sweats; chills; nausea or vomiting.

If you suffer from severe allergic reactions to any insect or spider bite or sting, a doctor can prescribe an **arthropod anaphylactic kit** which you should keep with you. This kit is intended to begin to manage a severe reaction and give you time to get to a healthcare facility. It *does not* substitute for going to the hospital.

Some venoms, such as that of some rattlesnakes, cause so much tissue damage that any allergic reactions are secondary until the venom is neutralized or has run its course.

When a person has been bitten or stung by any animal there is always the chance of infection and the area should be thoroughly cleaned with soap and water and an antiseptic applied to kill any germs that were on the stinger or teeth of the animal. If there is much pain, an ice cube applied to the wound for a short period should help. Do not leave the ice cube on for more than one minute at a time. A mild pain reliever can also be taken if necessary.

If there is a puncture wound left from the bite or sting and you have not had a tetanus booster shot in the last five years please consult a physician.

SCORPIONS

Centruroides exilicauda, Vejovis spinigeris, Hadrurus arizonensis

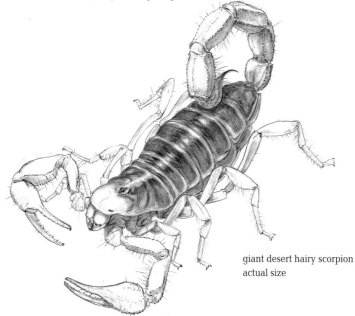

giant desert hairy scorpion
actual size

Description ♦ Scorpions are an integral part of the ecosystems they inhabit and their propensity for consuming large quantities of plant-eating insects has won them grudging respect from farmers around the world. Though scorpions are reputed to be among the deadliest inhabitants of our desert regions, of the thirty species represented in Arizona the sting of only one—the **bark scorpion** (*Centruroides exili-cauda*)—is regarded as life threatening. The bark scorpion averages one to one and one-half inches in length and is usually light tan in color. Its slender pincers and tail distinguish it from its less toxic cousins; at its widest, its body will not exceed one-fourth inch. Unlike other scorpions, it is often found clinging to the underside of its hiding place.

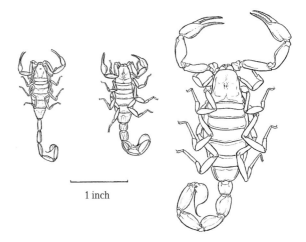

1 inch

Less dangerous are the **striped tail scorpion** (*Vejovis spinigeris*), one and one-half inches in length with a heavier body than the bark scorpion and usually darker in color and with a striped tail; and the **giant desert hairy scorpion** (*Hadrurus arizonensis*), five and one-half inches in length and pale yellow in color.

Habitat ✦ The **bark scorpion**, as its name implies, is usually associated with trees and is the only Arizona species that does not burrow. It can be found in riparian and other wooded areas, in moist microhabitats under bark, boards, plants, and fallen tree litter. In urban and suburban settings it is most likely to be found in newly disturbed areas.

The **striped tail scorpion** and **giant desert hairy scorpion** are often known as "ground scorpions" and in the desert can be found in lumber piles, under rocks, in cracks, and in moist places.

Scorpions are nocturnal creatures and are rarely seen during daylight hours or during the winter months.

Prevention ✦ Because **bark scorpions** can hang upside down on most surfaces, use caution when picking up rocks, boards, or other debris. Scorpions are not aggressive toward humans. When in scorpion habitat, shake out and visually inspect all clothing, bedding, and shoes before use, as stings frequently occur when the scorpion has been trapped in these articles. Make sure doors and windows are tight fitting with good weather stripping, and that any other openings are closed or fitted with a fine mesh screen. Keep houses and yards free of clutter and debris, and handle firewood and building materials with care. Because of the scorpion's secretive nature, no control measures would be effective or wanted.

Delivery of venom and symptoms ✦ The venom injecting apparatus of the scorpion is located in the tail or telson. At the tip of the telson are the venom gland, venom reservoir, and stinger. The telson tip is brought up and over the body to sting whatever is being grasped in the pincers.

The venom of the **bark scorpion** contains many neurotoxins and causes immediate and severe pain at the sting site but very little inflammation or swelling. There will be tingling or a prickly feeling at the sting site. Further reactions to the venom include restlessness progressing to convulsions, slurred speech, drooling, muscle twitches and respiratory difficulties. These symptoms usually subside within twenty-four to seventy-two hours.

Stings of non-lethal species will produce localized pain at the sting site, a little swelling, and some discoloration of the surrounding tissues that usually lasts for no more than four to six hours.

Treatment ✦ **Scorpion stings can be life threatening. Contact a doctor or a local poison control center in all suspected cases of scorpion envenomation.**

Children, the elderly, and people with respiratory problems are most likely to have life threatening reactions to bark scorpion stings and should receive medical examination and observation.

Ninety-five percent of all scorpion stings can be treated at home *with the guidance of a healthcare professional.* Clean the wound with soap and water. To reduce pain, apply ice directly to the sting site for a brief period and take a mild analgesic such as aspirin or acetaminophen.

See page 32 for discussion of allergic reactions and recommended responses.

GIANT DESERT CENTIPEDE

Scolopendra heros

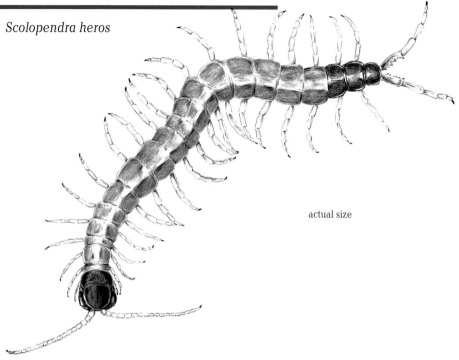

actual size

Description ◆ The giant desert centipede averages eight inches in length, but can be twelve inches long. Its body is light orange to yellowish in color. The head and tail are both darker, perhaps an adaption to confuse predators about which end to grab; choose the wrong one and experience a painful bite. Giant centipedes have an average of twenty body segments and, as in all centipedes, each segment has one pair of legs.

Habitat ◆ Centipedes dwell outdoors in dark, moist areas, under rocks, boards, and debris; and indoors they can be found in basements, closets, and garages of houses situated in or near the desert. Desert centipedes are active year round and hunt insects and other small creatures during warm winter days and summer nights.

Prevention ◆ Be careful where you put your hands and feet. If you see a centipede, do not pick it up, just watch and enjoy. Make sure doors and windows are tight fitting with good weather stripping, and that any other openings are closed or fitted with a fine mesh screen.

Delivery of venom and symptoms ◆ The giant desert centipede has large, pincerlike jaws that can inflict a nasty bite which, while painful, is not a serious injury. The venom, a cytolysin, dissolves cells and can cause localized pain and some inflammation. The pain can persist for days and the wound may produce pus.

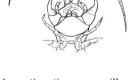

Treatment ◆ Simply keep the wound clean with soap and water. An antiseptic cream will help ward off infection. A tetanus shot is advisable for all puncture wound victims. Any discomfort can usually be treated with a mild pain reliever.

See page 32 for discussion of allergic reactions and recommended responses.

TARANTULA

Aphonopelma spp., *Dugesiella* spp.

actual size

Description ♦ These gentle giants are the largest spiders in the Southwest deserts. The term tarantula refers to all spiders in the family Theraphosidae. Arizona has approximately thirty species in the genera *Aphonopelma* and *Dugesiella*. Adults vary in size with leg span from two to four inches and are generally light to dark brown with dense hair on the abdomen and legs.

The tarantula hawk preys upon the tarantula by stinging and paralyzing it. The wasp then lays her eggs on it and her young are sustained with abundant and fresh food.

Habitat ♦ Our southwestern tarantulas live in burrows in open, undisturbed areas of the desert, where they spend their days resting and digesting. They hunt at night, rarely venturing more than a few yards from their burrows, preying mainly on large insects. A female tarantula will live her entire life, up to twenty years, in one burrow which she dug as a spiderling and enlarged as necessary. The male lives in his burrow for up to ten years before he reaches sexual maturity, then abandons it and commences to wander, sometimes great distances, in search of a female for reproduction. This movement usually occurs in June, July, and August, and humans most often come in contact with them during this period.

Prevention ♦ Most tarantula bites occur when people are molesting the creature in some way. These beautiful fellow inhabitants of the desert should be treated with respect.

Delivery of venom and symptoms ♦ Tarantulas employ two defensive strategies when confronted by a predator. They will rise up on their hind legs and bare their fangs, or they may rise up on their front legs and with their hind legs rapidly brush a cloud of fine urticating hairs off the abdomen toward their attacker. These hairs may be barbed and/or venomous and can cause severe itching and sores in mammals. Tarantula venom, delivered with a bite, is mild and there have been no severe envenomations recorded from our desert species. Symptoms should last less than twenty-four hours.

Treatment ♦ Being bitten by a tarantula or coming in contact with the urticating hairs, while sometimes painful, should not be cause for alarm. Urticating hairs may be removed from the skin surface with tape. Windblown urticating hairs can be swallowed or land in the eyes, and in this event, contact your local poison control center. If bitten, let the wound bleed freely for a few minutes and wash it with soap and water. A tetanus shot is advisable for all puncture wound victims.

See page 32 for discussion of allergic reactions and recommended responses.

BLACK WIDOW SPIDER

Latrodectus hesperus

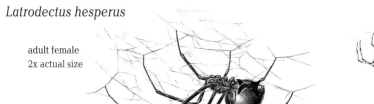

adult female
2x actual size

immature
spider

Description ✦ A very common and cosmopolitan spider, the black widow is small (usually about 3/8 inch long, with a leg span of one inch), and can also be dark brown in color; juveniles are patterned with red, brown, and beige. The black widow can be readily identified by a red hourglass marking on the female's abdomen, especially visible when she is in the web. The male, much smaller and brown colored, is too small to deliver a bite that penetrates the skin.

Habitat ✦ Female black widows rarely leave their webs. In the desert, these irregularly shaped structures are found in crevices, rodent burrows, and rock and debris piles. The preferred habitat for the black widow, though, seems to be manmade dwellings, and they build their webs in dark areas of garages, basements, and in firewood stacks, discarded cans, or unused equipment. They may be active indoors through the winter.

Prevention ✦ The black widow, although a ferocious predator, does not seek out or want to bite humans and most envenomations occur when the spider has been trapped, either by accident or when being molested. Make sure doors and windows are tight fitting with good weather stripping, and that any other openings are closed or fitted with a fine mesh screen. Keep houses and yards free of clutter, watch where you put your hands, and never harass a spider.

Delivery of venom and symptoms ✦ The venom of the black widow is produced in a pair of glands located in the cephalothorax and connected to fangs which are less than 1/50 inch long. The venom is a neuromuscular toxin and can cause muscle cramping beginning at the bite site, and in severe cases, respiratory problems, giddiness or nausea. Additional symptoms may include a pinprick pain at the bite site, and dull and progressive muscle pain which may spread from the bitten limb to other extremities. Symptoms may progress to muscular rigidity in the abdomen, shoulders, back, or chest. Other symptoms commonly reported include respiratory problems, restlessness, anxiety, nausea, vomiting, high blood pressure, headache, dizziness, and weakness. Severe symptoms should subside within twelve to twenty-four hours.

Treatment ✦ **Children, the elderly, people with high blood pressure, or persons suffering from other illness should see a doctor as quickly as possible.**

The majority of healthy adults can be treated at home *with the assistance of a local poison control center*, and should be given basic first aid to comfort them—mild pain relievers, a cool compress at the site of the bite, and a soak in a warm tub to relieve muscle cramping. Elevate the bitten limb to heart level.

See page 32 for discussion of allergic reactions and recommended responses.

BROWN RECLUSE SPIDER

Loxosceles arizonica, Loxosceles deserta

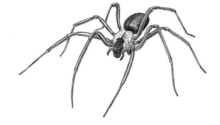

adult female
2x actual size

Description ♦ Brown recluse spiders average 5/16 inch in body length with a leg span of up to one inch. They vary in color from medium brown to tan. On the cephalothorax of the brown recluse spider there is a distinct violin-shaped marking pointing to the rear of the spider.

There are many brown spiders in the desert Southwest and, although closely related to the brown recluse spider (*Loxosceles reclusa*), our endemic spiders in the genus *Loxosceles* are not true recluse spiders, and their venom is less potent but still can be dangerous to humans.

Habitat ♦ The brown spiders of the desert Southwest seem to prefer dry, non-irrigated areas. They normally reside under logs, rocks, and debris, and in packrat nests and other similar habitats, where they spin heavy, irregular webs. In desert-situated buildings the brown spider may be found in bedding, clothing, and dark, unused corners. The brown spider searches for prey by night and sits in its web during the day. Although usually not active in the winter, they can be found out on warm days and in warm houses.

Prevention ♦ Brown spiders are not in any way aggressive toward humans and most bites occur when the spider is trapped in clothing, bedding or against some substrate. Watchfulness and basic precautions—shaking and checking bedding and clothes before use and looking before putting your hand under or into something—best prevent contact with brown recluse spiders. To control any spider population, keep debris and litter away from your house and yard. Make sure doors and windows are tight fitting with good weather stripping, and that any other openings are closed or fitted with a fine mesh screen.

Delivery of venom and symptoms ♦ The venom is injected through very small fangs, and most severe envenomations occur when people are bitten on a thin-skinned, fatty area such as the abdomen or thigh. In most instances little or no pain is felt, and in some cases people do not know they have been bitten. Within two to eight hours local pain and swelling along with flulike symptoms (fever, nausea, joint pain, vomiting) may appear. The venom is composed of enzymes that cause tissue breakdown, and within twelve hours to several days a necrotic lesion resembling a bulls-eye forms that can take months to heal. Fatal or near fatal envenomations are very rare.

Treatment ♦ **If you think that you have been bitten by a brown spider (genus *Loxosceles*, marked with a violin on its back), seek treatment from a physician or emergency room immediately.**

CONENOSE BUG

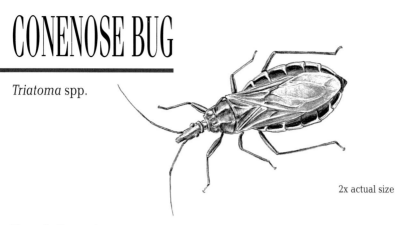

Triatoma spp.

2x actual size

Description ✦ Conenose bugs, members of the assassin bug family, Reduviidae, are parasitic insects that live on vertebrate blood and can be serious pests. The species that occur in the Southwest resemble one another in color, brown to black with orange checks along the margin of the wings and along the back. They are elongated in body shape, with distinctive neck and conical head. Their size varies from one-half inch to one inch.

Habitat ✦ City residents should rarely come in contact with conenose bugs because they are primarily parasites of packrats, which generally live in undisturbed desert areas. Residential lights on the outskirts of town and in desert areas attract them. When daylight comes, they must find a place to hide and many gain entrance into houses. Once inside, they hide wherever they can—in furniture, bedding, under carpeting— and at night come out to feed. Conenose bugs can be active almost year round but are most active during warm months.

Prevention ✦ Insecticides work in two ways: first by poisoning insects as it contacts their bodies, and second by eliminating the food source for bugs that eat other bugs. They are not effective in controlling conenose bugs because, being parasites living on mammalian blood, these insects do not depend on other insects for food; and applying these deadly chemicals to their hiding places, typically your bed and bedroom, would expose you to their poisons as well. If you suspect that you are living near large conenose bug populations, make sure doors and windows are tight fitting with good weather stripping, and that any other openings are closed or fitted with a fine mesh screen. The safest way to eradicate them once they have entered your home is to physically search them out: strip beds and check on and in between mattresses and blankets, remove everything from closet floors, carefully examine the carpet, check under furniture.

Delivery of venom and symptoms ✦ Conenose bugs bite their prey, then draw out the blood. They do not have venom producing glands per se, but their saliva glands produce enzymes that numb the area of the bite and stop the coagulation of blood while the conenose bug is feeding. Local reactions can appear, including pain, redness, swelling, and itching. If only mild local reactions occur, in a matter of hours the symptoms should disappear. Severe allergic reactions can develop when the victim has been sensitized by previous bites.

Treatment ✦ In the case of mild, local symptoms, wash the bite site with soap and water and apply an antiseptic ointment. If the pain is severe, a mild pain reliever can be taken.

See page 32 for discussion of allergic reactions and recommended responses.

PUSS CATERPILLAR

Megalopyge bissesa

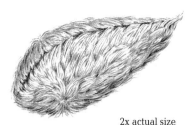

2x actual size

Description ◆ The puss caterpillar is the caterpillar stage of the flannel moth, which lays its eggs in trees and shrubs in spring or early summer; the eggs hatch within a few days and the caterpillars feed through the summer, pupate in cocoons over winter, and emerge in the spring as large (one and three-fourths inch) moths, with white and tan wings. Puss caterpillars grow to about one inch, have long "hairs" covering their bodies, and are dirty white to tan in coloration before they pupate.

Habitat ◆ Puss caterpillars can be found in riparian areas where deciduous trees, especially oak, and brush are abundant. They are active from early spring through the summer.

Prevention ◆ Instruct children not to play with puss caterpillars and avoid locations where they are seen. Usually no control is necessary because their numbers are kept in check by parasitic insects.

Delivery of venom and symptoms ◆ The long, silky hairs of the puss caterpillar hide black-tipped venom spines or urticating hairs. Envenomation occurs when an urticating hair, through which venom from a one-celled gland at the base of the hair can be injected by capillary action, pierces the victim's skin. The venom causes itching, pain, burning, and welting at the site. Symptoms may increase in severity for several hours and take several days to dissipate entirely. Wind-blown urticating hairs can be swallowed or land in the eyes. If this happens, contact your local poison control center.

Treatment ◆ For stings with no severe symptoms remove any hairs with tape, wash the affected area with soap and water, and apply ice to relieve the burning. A mild analgesic can be taken to relieve pain. Puss caterpillar stings vary in intensity.

See page 32 for discussion of allergic reactions and recommended responses.

ANTS, WASPS, AND BEES

Hymenoptera

These are the stinging and biting insects of the order Hymenoptera, the membrane-winged insects. They are prolific pollinators of flowering plants, including many crop plants, and some prey on plant-damaging insects. Studies of this group of social insects have provided important clues to our own behavior. They cause more human deaths every year—about 150—than all other venomous animals combined, probably because of their huge numbers and the benign regard afforded them by humans. Watchfulness and common sense will keep you away from these pesky yet useful insects.

harvester ants
2x actual size

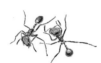

velvet ant
2x actual size

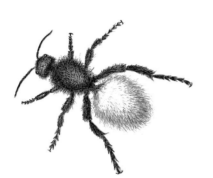

ANTS

Description and habitat ♦ The ants (family Formicidae), are abundant in the world with many species inhabiting many different ecological niches. The three genera of venomous ants in the southwestern United States are the **fire ants** (*Solenopsis* spp.), the **harvester ants** (*Pogonomyrmex* spp.) and the **field ants** (*Formica* spp.).

   Fire ants are 1/16 to 1/4 inch in size, dull yellow to red or black in color, and have fine hair on the head and abdomen; their legs are long. They are found in fields, woodlands, and open areas with dry to moist soil.

   Harvester ants, reddish brown in color and 1/4 to 1/2 inch long, live in cultivated fields, bare areas, and sandy areas near roadways.

   Field ants, can be black and red, or just black, or just red, or even brown and are 1/16 to 1/4 inch long. They occur in a variety of habitats, including mountainous areas and are common in houses both in the desert and urban areas.

Prevention ♦ There are many commercial ant-specific insecticides available to control ants that have become a serious nuisance. All insecticides should be used carefully and kept away from children, pets, and open water. Seal all possible entry points to keep ants out of your house.

Delivery of venom and symptoms ♦ All ants bite defensively, but **fire ants** and **harvester ants** also inject their victims with venom located in the stinger, causing severe pain and blistering. The pain should subside rather quickly and the blistering should heal within a day or two. Repeated exposure to the venoms of the fire and harvester ants can cause sensitization.

The **field ant** bites its victim then, from glands located in the rear of the ant, sprays formic acid on the wound. The formic acid causes short-lived although sometimes severe pain, usually with no other symptoms.

Treatment ◆ If symptoms are mild with only localized pain and/or blistering, keep the wound clean with soap and water and apply an antiseptic.

See page 32 for discussion of allergic reactions and recommended responses.

WASPS

Description and habitat ◆ Wasps are a large group that include **velvet ants** (family Mutillidae), **spider wasps** (family Pompilidae), **umbrella wasps** and **yellowjackets**, also known as hornets (family Vespidae), and **mud daubers** (family Sphecidae).

Velvet ants, are actually wingless wasps. They vary in size from one-fifth to one inch, and parasitize ground-nesting wasps and bees by laying their eggs on the pupae of the host. They are furry and brightly colored in black and red, yellow, or orange. They live in open, undisturbed desert areas and are infrequent visitors in desert houses.

Spider wasps are sometimes large (up to one and one-half inch), glossy blue-black, solitary insects. They live in underground burrows and prey upon spiders. There are many species of spider wasps in the southwestern United States. The tarantula hawk is the largest spider wasp and, of course, preys upon the largest spider, the tarantula.

Umbrella or **paper wasps** are large (averaging three-fourths inch) and are usually dull yellow or brown with a tapering mid-body. These social animals build hanging, umbrella-shaped nests of a paper-like substance in palm trees, shrubbery and under eaves in man-made structures, stock them with insect prey, and defend them quite vigorously. When a potential predator (humans included) nears the nest a guard wasp displays a warning. If this is not heeded, worker wasps attack.

Yellowjackets, as their name implies, are marked with bands of black and yellow and average about one-half inch in length. They nest in the ground or in fallen logs. Not quite as aggressive as umbrella wasps they will defend their nest or a food source (such as a soda or hamburger at a picnic) with pugnacity.

Mud daubers are solitary wasps of medium size (one-half inch in length), dark blue, black, or green with a very thin, stalk-like midbody. Under rocks, overhanging cliffs, or roofs, they build small mud nests which they provision with paralyzed spiders to feed their young. Mud daubers are not aggressive even when guarding their nest and are reported to have a relatively harmless sting.

Prevention ◆ **Mud daubers, yellowjackets,** and **umbrella wasps** all build nests near or on human dwellings and caution should be used when working in your yard or trying to remove nests. If you need to remove a nest, call a pest control expert or your county extension agency for information.

Velvet ants and **spider wasps** are rarely encountered in human habitations. Do not disturb or molest them and they will leave you alone.

Delivery of venom and symptoms ◆ Both **velvet ants** and **spider wasps** have powerful venom delivered by a sting, but are not aggressive towards humans and should not be considered a threat. Stings usually occur when they have either been stepped on or molested in some way. Symptoms of the sting include sometimes severe localized pain and usually the formation of a small welt. The pain should subside rather quickly and the welt should heal within a day or two.

   Umbrella wasps sting with an unbarbed stinger which can be used repeatedly. Symptoms of the sting include sometimes severe localized pain and usually the formation of a small welt. The pain should subside rather quickly and the welt should heal within a day or two.

   The **yellowjacket** stinger is unbarbed and can be inserted many times causing considerable pain. Symptoms of the sting include sometimes severe localized pain and usually the formation of a small welt. The pain should subside rather quickly and the welt should heal within a day or two.

   The **mud daubers** are usually very calm and are not known for a painful sting.

Treatment ◆ People can become sensitized to the venom of any of these insects. For a sting that is causing no threatening reactions, use soap and water to clean the wound and apply an antiseptic. It has been reported that a baking soda or meat tenderizer paste may reduce the pain, and antihistamines can reduce other mild symptoms. The pain should subside quickly, and it is only necessary to keep the wound clean and aseptic.

See page 32 for discussion of allergic reactions and recommended responses.

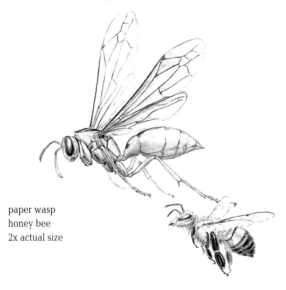

paper wasp
honey bee
2x actual size

BEES

Description ◆ Bees (family Apidae) are among the most important plant pollinators and also among the most significant venomous animals. In some species, each female lives and broods larvae in a nesting tunnel which may be underground or in wood. Honey bees and bumblebees live in colonies and are the only bees to produce and store honey. Honey bees, though not native to the United States, have become widespread, with both domestic and escaped wild populations.

   In defending the hive, bees employ swarming behavior that drives away predators. This behavior infrequently involves humans because the domesticated and wild honey bees we come in contact with most often are descendent from European bees bred to be non-aggressive.

   A more aggressive africanized bee has recently made an appearance in the south-western United States. The africanized bee's venom is no stronger than our common honey bee's. What makes them dangerous is their aggressive instinct to swarm in large numbers and sting, sometimes thousands of times, whatever or whomever they perceive as a threat. Massive numbers of stings may introduce a lethal dose of venom. The africanized bee poses the greatest hazard to farmers and beekeepers along its path of travel following riparian corridors and irrigated lands (agricultural and land-scaped) into the United States. Interbreeding with domesticated bees, upon which farmers depend to pollinate their crops and from which beekeepers collect honey, results in bees that are not as productive. Africanized bees can be distinguished from the common honey bees of the United States only through careful analysis of certain body parts by a qualified entomologist.

Habitat ✦ Most bees are solitary and nest in burrows and crevices in the ground, in plants, and sometimes in buildings. Honey bees build hives in hollow trees and hives provided by beekeepers. Bumblebee colonies are underground.

Prevention ✦ Because the domesticated bee cannot be distinguished easily from the africanized bee, avoid all bees. Bee hives or swarms should be removed only by pest control experts. Contact your local poison control center for the names of qualified bee removal specialists.

Delivery of venom and symptoms ✦ Because bees are strictly nectar feeders, their venom has evolved not to paralyze but to be painful and is very distressing to mammals. Venom is delivered through a modified ovi-depositor, which is in the stinger on the rear of the bee. The venom of social bees, while painful, is usually mild unless a person has become sensitized by repeated stings or is allergic to bee venom. Normal symptoms of the sting include sometimes severe localized pain and usually the formation of a small welt.

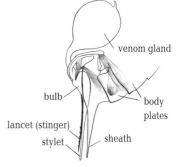

Treatment ✦ If you are stung by a **single bee**, simply clean the site with soap and water and apply an antiseptic. It has been reported that a baking soda or meat tenderizer paste may reduce the pain, and antihistamines can reduce other mild symptoms. If you are **swarmed** protect your eyes and face and try to get away and seek help. **If you are stung multiple times or are experiencing unusual or severe symptoms because of a single sting get medical assistance immediately.**

See page 32 for discussion of allergic reactions and recommended responses.

RATTLESNAKES

Crotalus spp., *Sistrurus catenatus*

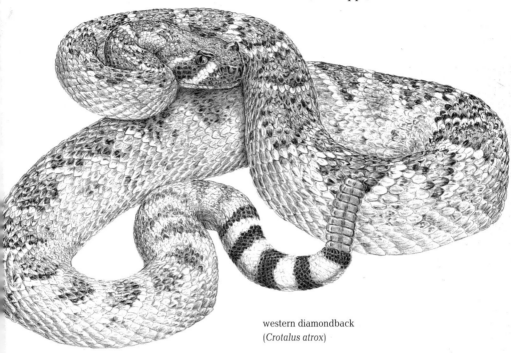

western diamondback
(*Crotalus atrox*)

Description ♦ Rattlesnakes, exclusively New World animals, originated in middle America. There are thirteen species of rattlesnakes in the western United States in two genera, *Crotalus* and *Sistrurus*. They, along with the copperhead and water moccasin, both of the genus *Agkistrodon*, of Texas and points east, are pit vipers, so named because located between each eye and nostril they have a small, heat-sensing pit. Other distinguishing features of rattlesnakes include the flattened, triangular head; some sort of rattle, whether it is a prebutton or a remnant; elliptical pupils (cat's eyes); and, seen only when it's too late, foldable fangs. Rattlesnakes are heavily built and range from under thirty inches to over sixty inches in length and are cryptically colored, usually in tans and browns but can be orange, red, bright green, yellow, black or peach. Most are mottled or banded, with lighter underside.

The rattle is composed of hollow segments of keratin, the same substance of which human hair and fingernails are composed. Many different snakes vibrate their tail as a defensive or warning display. The rattle has evolved to give full effect, possibly as a response to the large populations of predators and hoofed animals once present throughout the Americas. It is especially effective in warning its most dangerous predators, humans. Do not rule out a rattlesnake identification based on the absence of rattles though; an entire rattle or part of it may be missing. Young have only a small prebutton and really cannot rattle until their first or second shed when a new segment is added. The Catalina Island rattlesnake from Isla Catalina in the Gulf of California lacks rattles altogether.

Rattlesnakes will enter buildings, disturbed areas, and irrigated areas (golf courses, gardens, etc.) in search of shelter and food, and prey upon a diverse selection of food items: Larger snakes prey on rabbits, wood rats, and birds; smaller ones will eat small rodents, lizards, and amphibians. Rattlesnakes will sit and wait or actively search for prey. When a warm-blooded target is found, the snake quickly bites and lets go, then follows, using heat and scent trails, till the prey animal succumbs to the venom. When it bites a cold-blooded animal, the rattlesnake holds on till its venom takes effect.

Rattlesnakes are preyed upon by many different animals: badgers, hawks, coyotes, roadrunners, and other snakes to name a few. Kingsnakes have been known to eat very large rattlesnakes, and apparently have some immunity to their venom.

Habitat ♦ They are found throughout the United States in a variety of habitats, but the deserts and mountains of the Southwest seem to be havens for rattlesnake species. Rattlesnakes are active at night during the hot summers and during the day in the warm spring, winter, and fall days. They inhabit many areas where the potential for human-rattlesnake interaction is high, including recreation areas, homes, and businesses that are adjacent to undisturbed or newly disturbed desert areas and farmland.

Prevention ♦ When humans move into desert areas the rate of rattlesnake encounters rises, especially in newly disturbed areas where populations of snakes are in flux. In these areas, numbers of snakes will settle to new, lower levels, and encounters should decline, but even in areas with decreased natural habitat the chance for rattlesnake encounters is present. To minimize the likelihood of meeting a rattlesnake in or around your house, seal all possible entry ways into your house and garage, seal or fill all possible snake hiding or nesting areas—holes and cracks under rocks, trees and foundations—and keep your yard clean and clutter-free. There is no way if you have a landscaped yard to eliminate all places where a snake could lay up, but you can reduce those areas. Remove packrat nests from your property as humanely as possible. Be careful where you put your feet and hands and keep a sharp eye when hiking. If you encounter a rattlesnake, give it a wide berth and time to leave before you walk in the same area again. If you come upon one near your house, give it time to leave (most snakes will just be passing through); if you have repeated encounters, call your local poison control center for information on removing them.

According to local experts up to 75 percent of all rattlesnake bites are illegitimate, meaning that the snakes were being harassed or, in some cases, kept as pets when the bite occurred. Leave rattlers alone and they will leave you alone. Rattlesnakes will not chase or attack anything they cannot swallow, and will bite only when cornered or as a last resort.

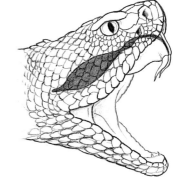

Delivery of venom and symptoms ♦ Venom is produced in two glands that duct directly into a pair of hypodermic fangs that fold up and out of the way when not in use. These fangs are needle sharp and can be an inch long. Rattlesnake venom, which is complex and varies in makeup and strength from species to species, is hemotoxic, and with the Mohave rattlesnake also neurotoxic. It can cause severe tissue damage and is potentially life threatening. When venom is injected, symptoms appear quickly, and include swelling and intense pain, and as time progresses chills and weakness, pulse and respiratory irregularities, numbness in the face, nausea, and then bleeding and sloughing of tissue. Most of these symptoms can be reduced or avoided with the use of an antivenin.

Some doctors and herpetologists believe that in up to 25 percent of all rattlesnake bites no venom is injected.

Treatment ♦ First aid for rattlesnake bite victims is simple: **Transport to the nearest hospital without delay.** Keep the bite victim calm, warm, and comfortable. **Do not** apply a tourniquet, administer any drugs or alcohol, apply ice or attempt any other first aid such as cut-and-suck or electroshock. These will waste time and will cause more harm than good. A tetanus shot is advisable for all puncture wound victims.

People who anticipate being in areas where transport to a hospital could be delayed more than half a day should contact their local poison control center in advance of their trip for first aid information.

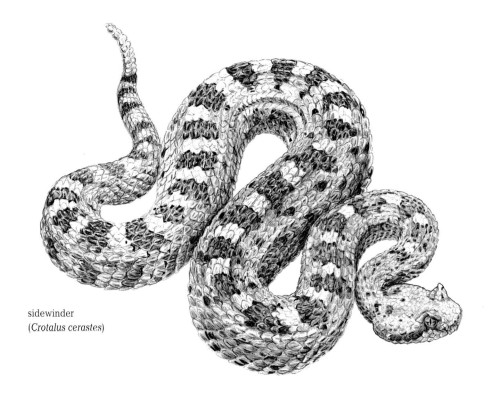

sidewinder
(*Crotalus cerastes*)

ARIZONA CORAL SNAKE

Micruroides euryxanthus

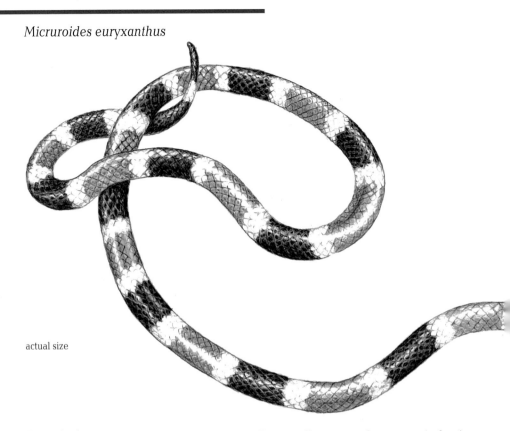

actual size

Description ✦ The Arizona coral snake is small, generally no more than twenty inches in length and about as big around as a finger. It is a relative of the larger and more venomous eastern coral snake (*Micurus fulvius*), and both belong to the family Elapidae, which also includes the cobras and the African mamba. Prominent black, yellow, and red bands encircle its body. The sequential pattern of colors—black head followed by bands of yellow/red/yellow/black—distinguishes the coral snake. A simple rhyme may be helpful in remembering what to watch for: Red on yellow kill a fellow; red on black venom lack.

    Some non-venomous snakes have mimicked the bright coloration of the coral snake as protection from predators. Imitators have black and red bands touching, or the bands do not encircle the body. These include the long-nosed snake (*Rhinocheilus lecontei*), some king and milk snakes (*Lampropeltis* spp.), and the shovel-nosed snakes (*Chionactis* spp.).

Habitat ✦ In their range, across southern Arizona and southwestern New Mexico, Arizona coral snakes live underground in rocky undisturbed desert highlands, forests, and canyons and are rarely seen. They are active at night during warm weather and sometimes during warm winter days.

Prevention ✦ As with all snakes, the Arizona coral snake is much more afraid of you than you should be of it, and will bite only as a last resort. It is passive and will hide its head in its coil and vibrate its tail to draw the attention of a predator away from more vital areas of its body. No snake, especially the Arizona coral snake, will sneak up and bite you. Their venom is for subduing and digesting prey and is expensive to produce and, therefore, not readily wasted on large animals. This beautiful snake should not be molested in any way but enjoyed from a safe distance.

Delivery of venom and symptoms ♦ The venom is produced in two glands in the snake's head and is channeled to two grooved fangs that deliver the venom while the snake hangs on to its prey. The venom, a neurotoxin, while not as strong as the eastern coral snake's is still two to three times stronger than that of the western diamondback rattlesnake. Because of its small mouth and non-aggressive nature, very few envenomations have ever occurred. In the cases of bites reported, careless handling of the snake was involved. Symptoms, if any, appear within one to two hours and consist of a little pain and numbness, drowsiness, weakness, and giddiness. There usually is no swelling or redness at the site of the bite.

Treatment ♦ First aid for bite victims is simple: If you are bitten by an Arizona coral snake **seek medical help immediately** and remain calm. Keep warm, and comfortable. **Do not** apply a tourniquet, administer any drugs or alcohol, or attempt any other first aid such as cut-and-suck or electroshock. These will waste time and will cause more harm than good. A tetanus shot is advisable for all puncture wound victims.

People who anticipate being in areas where transport to a hospital could be delayed more than a half a day should contact their local poison control center for first aid information in advance of their trip.

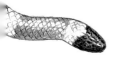

REAR FANGED SNAKES

Family Colubridae

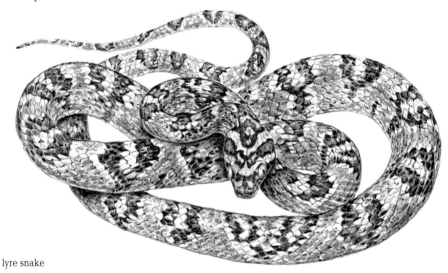

lyre snake

The family Colubridae, which includes rear fanged snakes, is the largest group of snakes, comprising 70 percent of all snake species worldwide. Most are non-venomous and include king and milk snakes, rat and corn snakes, and pine and gopher snakes. There are at least ten snake species in the desert Southwest that have enlarged rear teeth and some sort of venom-producing glands. The **western hognose snake** (*Heterodon nasicus*); the **night snake** (*Hypsiglena torquata*); the **lyre snake** (*Trimorphodon biscutatus*); and the **black headed snake** (*Tantilla hobartsmithi*) are common rear fanged snakes that can bite humans, but none have venom of sufficient potency to be a serious threat. All are very shy and have elaborate defensive behaviors that do not involve biting. They prey upon small lizards, snakes, mammals, and amphibians, and usually are nocturnal.

Description and habitat ♦ The **western hognose** is a thickbodied snake that uses its turned up nose for burrowing. This snake is usually around two feet in length but can be longer, and is tan or brown in color with darker saddles and side blotches. It is found in a variety of habitats, but usually near riparian areas where it specializes in preying upon toads.

The **night snake** is small, usually eighteen inches long, with a distinct, almost triangular head, eyes with vertical pupils, and light brown to grey coloration with light saddles down the back and a darker blotch on the neck. Night snakes prefer dry habitats and can be found in desert foothills, scrublands, and grasslands.

The **lyre snake**, brown and tan in color, with hexagonal markings split with a light crossbar, is distinguished by a light lyre-shaped marking on its head. The snake is usually two to three feet in length and has an almost triangular head, and eyes with vertical pupils. Rock dwellers, they prefer arid or semi-arid habitat, and are excellent climbers in both rocks and trees.

The **black headed snake** is usually under a foot long and has a dark top of the head, a lighter collar, usually a brown or grayish body, and a red stripe on its belly. It lives in a variety of habitats from the mountains down to the desert floor and spends most of its time under rocks, downed vegetation, or in holes in the ground.

Prevention ◆ These snakes are beneficial to their environment, pose no threat to humans or domesticated animals, and are fascinating and beautiful to watch and study. They should never be molested, killed, or captured.

Delivery of venom and symptoms ◆ The rear fanged snakes have enlarged hind teeth that are used to grasp and hold, then envenomate their prey. The teeth are not hypodermic, but some are grooved to facilitate the introduction of venom into the wound. Not all rear fanged snakes possess venom-producing glands, and of the ones that do, none in the United States produce venom toxic enough to harm a human. A bite usually produces a small itch, a little redness, and swelling.

Treatment ◆ The symptoms should not last long and washing the bite with soap and water and keeping it clean and aseptic will prevent secondary infection. A tetanus shot is advisable for all puncture wound victims.

See page 32 for discussion of allergic reactions and recommended responses.

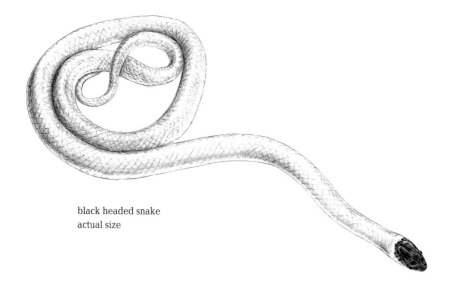

black headed snake
actual size

GILA MONSTER

Heloderma suspectum

Description ♦ Devil lizard or gentle desert dweller? The gila monster is one of the most misunderstood, maligned, molested, and mythologized animals in the world. Only recently have scientists begun to understand its biology. The gila monster is the largest lizard in the United States and one of only two venomous lizards in the world, the other being the closely related Mexican beaded lizard (*Heloderma horridum*), occurring in Mexico. The gila monster is a large and heavy lizard, up to twenty inches in length and two pounds in weight, and usually brightly colored in black with pink, yellow, or orange stripes or blotches. Its has a large head, a round body, and short and stubby legs. The tail, in which fat is stored, can be either plump and round or short and shriveled, depending on time of year and nutritional state of the lizard.

Habitat ♦ Gila monsters are fairly abundant in certain habitats, but are hardly ever seen. They spend more than 95 percent of their lives underground and are usually active above ground only in the spring and during summer monsoons. They are active during the daytime but occasionally can be found out on warm summer nights. They prefer desert foothills, where cover and prey are found easily within their very limited individual ranges.

Prevention ♦ Gila monsters are gentle desert lizards that take only what they need and flee from interaction with humans. Only when the lizard has been cornered or picked up will it try to bite. They sometimes wander into yards of houses that have been built in prime gila monster territory. If you are uneasy about a resident gila monster, call your local poison control center for advice.

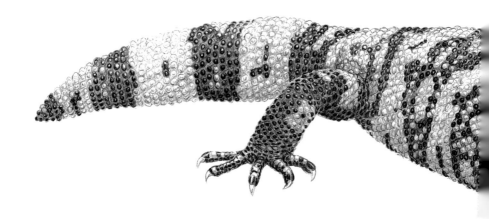

Delivery of venom and symptoms ♦ Since
gila monsters generally prey upon animals
that don't run or fight back—newborn and
young rabbits, birds and rodents—their
venom has evolved into a defensive rather
than offensive weapon, and it is extremely
painful and debilitating to potential
predators, including humans. Venom of
the gila monster is produced in glands
located in the lower jaw and is ducted to
the base of grooved teeth, resulting in a

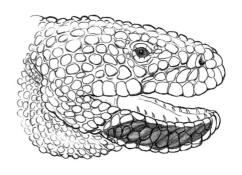

many-fanged bite. When a gila monster bites, it bites hard and does not let go; it
grinds its jaws to pump venom from the glands onto the teeth, causing an extremely
painful and sometimes ripped and torn bite wound. Usually its jaws must be pried
apart with a stick. Sometimes a glancing bite will occur and the lizard does not hang
on, but in any case a physician should be seen immediately. Symptoms of a gila
monster bite include intense pain, bleeding, swelling, low blood pressure and resulting
weakness. The pain will subside usually within a couple of hours and other symptoms
within five or six hours.

Treatment ♦ **In any case of gila monster bite a physician should be seen immediately** to
evaluate degree of envenomation and clean out the wound, which in many cases will
have teeth imbedded in it. A tetanus shot is advisable for all puncture wound victims.

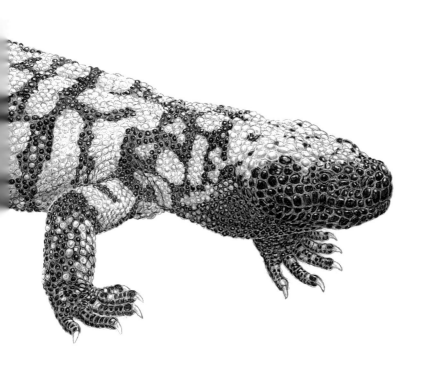

HARMLESS DESERT DWELLERS

By virtue of their appearance, some creatures of the Southwest deserts are thought to be venomous. Many of the non-venomous animals will consume and help control populations of many types of arthropods, some of which are venomous.

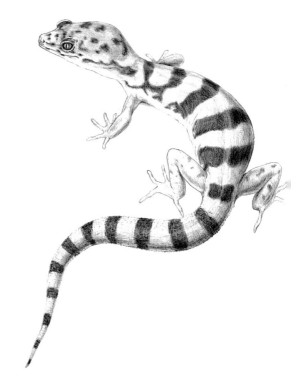

BANDED GECKO
Coleonyx variegatus

These inoffensive little creatures are sometimes mistaken for juvenile gila monsters. They are actually thin-skinned lizards that cannot control water loss as well as other desert lizards and can live in the desert only underground and be active only at night. They average two inches in length and are tan to yellow with brown bands along the back. They are non-venomous and prey upon arthropods. Many are seen near windows, where insects are drawn to lights at night, or in covered holes in the ground such as water meter boxes. They are quite tame.

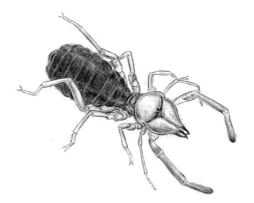

SOLPUGID
Eremobates spp.

The solpugid is also called the sun spider, and does indeed resemble a spider, its relative. It is usually about two inches in total length, brown in color, and quite hairy. It has very large and conspicuous jaws that can inflict a painful bite but it is non-venomous and not at all aggressive. Active both night and day in search of prey, they will venture into homes situated in the desert. Solpugids are ravenous eaters and can be beneficial in the control of venomous arthropods. If you are bitten by a solpugid, very unlikely unless you molest it, clean the bite with soap and water. Any pain will go away quickly.

28

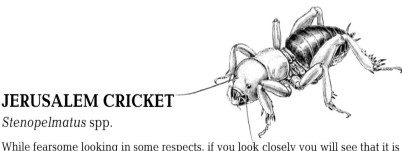

JERUSALEM CRICKET
Stenopelmatus spp.

While fearsome looking in some respects, if you look closely you will see that it is indeed only a cricket and crickets are not venomous. It can measure one and one-half inches in length and is quite robust. It is brown in color and some people say that if you look closely at the top of its head you can see a "smiley" face. Jerusalem crickets live under leaf litter, sand, and debris and are usually active only at night. While not venomous, if picked up or molested they can inflict a little bite that should not hurt at all.

VINEGAROON
Order Uropygi

This arthropod, while resembling a scorpion, lacks any venom injecting mechanism. Common throughout the southern half of the United States, it is usually active at night and rarely seen. The vinegaroon, or whip scorpion, can be up to three inches in length. It has a set of long front legs that are modified as feelers and a long, whiplike tail that is used to flail a stream of acetic acid toward any potential predator. If you are sprayed by a vinegaroon, wash the area thoroughly with soap and water. If you are sprayed in the eyes or mouth, rinse well with water.

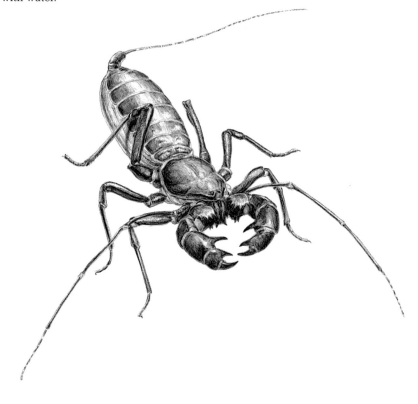

GLOSSARY

Analgesic—A drug that relieves pain, used here to mean a mild pain reliever such as aspirin or acetaminophen, never a narcotic or alcohol.

Anaphylactic shock—A severe and sometimes fatal allergic reaction to a foreign substance; example venom. Commonly characterized by troubled breathing and slowed heartbeat.

Antibiotic—A substance used to kill organisms, usually bacteria or viruses, that can cause infections.

Arachnid—Any of a class of arthropods comprising mostly air-breathing invertebrates, including spiders and scorpions, mites, and ticks, and having segmented bodies divided into two regions of which the anterior bears four pairs of legs. They have no antennae.

Arthropod—Any of a phylum of invertebrate animals (as insects, arachnids, and crustaceans) whose shared characteristics include a jointed body and limbs, and usually a shell which is molted at intervals.

Cephalothorax—The united head and thorax of an arachnid.

Cytolysin—A substance that dissolves cells.

Envenomation—The delivery of venom by a bite or sting.

Hemolysin—A substance that causes the dissolution of red blood cells.

Hypertension—Abnormally high blood pressure.

Hypotension—Abnormally low blood pressure.

Invertebrate—Lacking a spinal column.

Lesion—An abnormal change in structure of an organ or part due to injury.

Necrosis—Localized death of living tissue.

Neurotoxin—A poisonous protein complex that acts on the nervous system.

Ovi-depositor—The tubular or valved structure with which the eggs are placed.

Telson—The terminal segment of the body of an arthropod.

Tetanus—An acute infectious disease caused by the specific toxin of a bacillus (*Clostridium tetani*) which is usually introduced through a wound.

Urticating hair—A hollow, porous hair through which venom from a one-celled gland at the base can be injected by capillary action.

Venom—Poisonous matter secreted by some animals and transmitted to prey chiefly by biting or stinging.

Vertebrate—Having a spinal column.

REFERENCES

Banner, W. Jr. 1988. Bites and Stings in the Pediatric Patient. *Current Problems in Pediatrics.* Chicago: Year Book Medical.

Binder, L.S. 1989. Acute Arthropod Envenomation: Incidence, Clinical Features and Management. *Medical Toxicology, Adverse Drug Experience* 4:163–173.

Boyer, L. Hassen. 1991. Reptile and Arthropod Envenomations. *Occupational Medicine State of the Art Review* Vol. 6 No. 3:447–461

Dart, R.C., J.T. McNally, D.W. Spaite, and R. Gustafson. The Sequelae of Pitviper Poisoning in the United States. *Biology of the Pitvipers*, edited by Jonathan Campbell and E.D. Brodie, Jr. Tyler, TX: Felva, 1992.

Hunt, G.R. 1981. Bites and Stings of Uncommon Arthropods Part 2. *Postgraduate Medicine* Vol. 70 No. 2:107–114

Lowe C.H., C.R. Schwalbe, and T.B. Johnson. *The Venomous Reptiles of Arizona.* Phoenix: Nongame Branch Arizona Game and Fish Department, 1986.

McNally, J.T. Arizona Poison and Drug Information Center, Tucson. Personal communication regarding recommended first aid for venomous bites and stings, 1995.

The Moseby Medical Encyclopedia. New York: C.V. Moseby Co., 1985.

Schmidt, J.O. Carl Hayden Bee Laboratory, United States Department of Agriculture, Tucson, Arizona. Personal communication regarding africanized honey bee, 1995.

Smith, R.L. *Venomous Animals of Arizona.* Tucson: University of Arizona, Cooperative Extension College of Agriculture, 1992.

Stebbins, R.C. *A Field Guide to Western Reptiles and Amphibians.* Boston: Houghton Mifflin Company, 1966.

AUTHOR'S ACKNOWLEDGMENTS

To my wife, Janet, and Cassidy and Delaney. I love you.

To Jude McNally, Assistant director of the Arizona Poison and Drug Information Center. Thanks, mentor, for all your help.

To Sandra Scott. Thanks for your patience, suggestions, and help.

Trevor Hare, Tucson, Arizona, 1995.

ARTIST'S ACKNOWLEDGMENTS

Most of the drawings in this book are based upon observations of live animals. Although this is perhaps the best way to produce good animal drawings, numerous logistical difficulties accompany this method. Many of the animals depicted herein are fragile, secretive, or only seasonally active. Some are dangerous to handle, others are legally protected. Aside from the few that I collected, it was only with the help of others that I was able to make drawings of living individuals. Exceptionally generous were Randy Babb of Arizona Game and Fish; and Andy Holycross and Robert Reed, graduate students at Arizona State University. I am also grateful to the following people for assistance and encouragement: Linda Allison, Mike Douglas, Diana Hews, Larry Neinaber, Steve Norris, Steve Rissing, Peter Scott, and Jeanie Simmons, all of Arizona State University; Bruce Bohmke, Mike Demlong, and Bryan Starrett, all with the Phoenix Zoo; and Barney Tomberlin of Hitari Invertebrates. For five drawings, I relied heavily on the work of photographers George H.H. Huey, David W. Middleton, John F. Moore III, and Sherwin F. Wood.

Barbara Terkanian, Tempe, Arizona, 1995.

ALLERGIC REACTIONS

About 5 percent of people who are repeatedly bitten develop allergic reactions which fall into three basic types:

Type I: Anaphylactic response, the most severe allergic reaction. It will begin within one hour of envenomation and is most likely to include facial swelling, respiratory distress, and a life-threatening drop in blood pressure. *Emergency medical transportation is warranted. CALL 911.*

Type II: May begin within the first hour and differs from Type I reaction in that it is less severe and frequently initiates at the site of envenomation. Symptoms may progress for several hours and may persist for days. *Contact your local poison control center or your doctor.*

Type III: Reactions may be delayed for hours or even days. *Contact your local poison control center or your doctor.*

Allergic reactions may include:
Burning pain and itching at the site of the wound;
Itching on the palms of the hands, soles of the feet, neck and groin;
General body swelling;
Facial swelling;
Nettlelike rash over the body;
Labored breathing;
Intense pain;
High or low blood pressure;
Sweats, chills, nausea or vomiting.
♦
Some persons feel slight depression followed by quickening of the pulse. Others feel faint, weak, and nauseated.

In very severe allergic reactions, these symptoms may lead to anaphylactic shock and unconsciousness.

A note about anaphylactic kits: These kits are available, by prescription only, to individuals who suffer reactions to bites or stings. An anaphylactic kit will only *begin* to manage a severe reaction by buying you some time until you can get definitive treatment in a healthcare facility. They *do not* substitute for going to a hospital.